The Rulings of Health and Safety: And How to Deal with the Corona-virus (COVID-19)

According to the rulings of
Grand Ayatollah Sayyid Mohammed Taqi al-Modarresi

Biography of Grand Ayatollah Sayyid Mohammed Taqi al-Modarresi

Grand Ayatollah Sayyid Mohammed-Taqi al-Husayni al-Modarresi (Arabic: محمد تقي الحسيني المدرسي) born in 1945 is an Iraqi Shia *marja'* and political theorist.

Grand Ayatollah Sayyid Mohammed-Taqi al-Husayni al-Modarresi is the author of over 400 books on matters of theology, historiography, jurisprudence, philosophy, logic and social science.

The Anglican Centre in Rome has stated that *"Grand Ayatollah al-Modarresi is probably the second most senior Shia cleric after al-Sistani. His call for peace & human dignity is very significant."*

Grand Ayatollah Sayyid Mohammed-Taqi al-Husayni al-Modarresi was born into a distinguished Shia religious family in Karbala, Iraq. His father is Ayatollah Sayyid Mohammed-Kadhim al-Modarresi. His mother is the daughter of grand Ayatollah Sayyid Mahdi al-Shirazi. He is from the descendants of the Prophet Mohammed (sawa).

Grand Ayatollah Sayyid Mohammed-Taqi al-Husayni al-Modarresi began his religious education in the religious seminaries of Karbala, at the young age of 8. He studied under some of Karbala's most senior scholars such as Shaykh Mohammed al-Karbassi, Shaykh Jafar al-Rushti, Shaykh Yusuf al-Khurasani and his uncle, Sayyid Mohammed al-Shirazi.

Due to the rising pressures of the Bathists anti-Shia sentiment Grand Ayatollah Sayyid Mohammed-Taqi al-Husayni al-Modarresi emigrated to Kuwait in 1971. He settled there until 1979, after which he moved to Iran. With the overthrow of Saddam Hussein by American-led forces in 2003, Grand Ayatollah Sayyid Mohammed-Taqi al-Husayni al-Modarresi along with other Iran-based clerics returned to Iraq.

Grand Ayatollah Sayyid Mohammed-Taqi al-Husayni al-Modarresi was the first Shia religious leader to issue a call to popular resistance against ISIS, after its swift capture of large swathes of land in Iraq in June 2014. In his statement, Grand Ayatollah Sayyid Mohammed-Taqi al-Husayni al-Modarresi warned against the destruction of churches and temples belonging to all religions.

Grand Ayatollah Sayyid Mohammed-Taqi al-Husayni al-Modarresi made an official statement regarding the COVID-19 strain, saying that the people of Iraq should self-isolate, and utilize the month of Rajab, by performing the recommended prayers and supplications at home. He also stated that Muslim community needs to increase its faith in God, so that He may protect us from all evil. Grand Ayatollah Sayyid Mohammed-Taqi al-Husayni al-Modarresi also called for the Iraqi government to take up all measures to face this new viral strain, which threatens the lives of many today. He added, the Iraqi people are always willing to stand by its government and provide aid, as is seen in the Arbaeen pilgrimage.

Grand Ayatollah Sayyid Mohammed-Taqi al-Husayni al-Modaressi traveled to Bahrain in 2002 on an official visit, at the invitation of the Minister of Justice and Islamic Affairs, Abdullah bin Khalid Al Khalifa.

In December 2014, Grand Ayatollah Sayyid Mohammed-Taqi al-Husayni al-Modarresi was invited by the Pope to attend a summit of world religious leaders at the

Vatican. This made him the first Grand Ayatollah to have met the Pope.

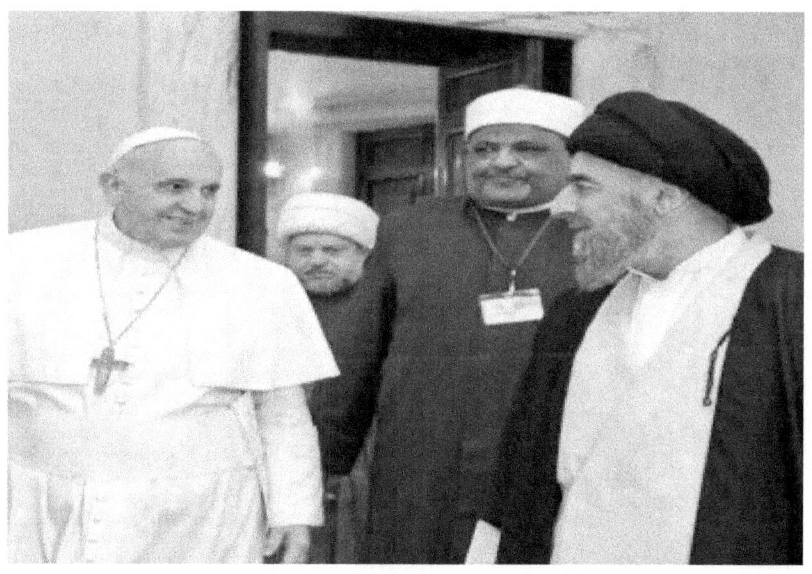

In his speech, Grand Ayatollah Sayyid Mohammed-Taqi al-Husayni al-Modarresi asked world religious leaders to "engage in a symbiosis of civilizations and religions". He condemned terrorism, nuclear proliferation, modern day slavery and said:

"At its core, divine religion is one, but failure to understand religion has divided human beings and created barriers between us. We must exert extra effort to tear down those barriers and join religions under the umbrella of a common term. We have a calling to love one another, to protect the environment, to stop the spread of weapons of mass destruction and to end slavery in all its forms."

In 2016 he went to Australia, where he met community leaders as well as the Australian Foreign Minister Julie Bishop. The two discussed Iraq, the war on terrorism, as well as how Muslims can be better integrated into the Australian community.[1]

---

[1] https://en.wikipedia.org/wiki/Mohammad_Taqi_al-Modarresi

In the Name of Allah, the Beneficent, the Merciful

Praise be to Allah, Lord of the Worlds, and may the blessings of Allah be upon Mohammed and his righteous Household. Whatever the source of this pandemic may be, it shows the serious weakness of the institutions of industrial countries, as they were unable to counter it.

If we look at it, it shows the deep weak points of our civilization which if we do not counter with all our ability, it may result in the collapse of our civil foundations. We will present to you, God-willing, a group of facts about this pandemic. Then we will mention some of the rulings of health and safety. Finally, some rulings regarding how to deal the COVID-19 pandemic, hoping it guides us all in our future challenges.

1. Is it a trial?

Humans in this world are subject to trial, whether as individuals or societies. Our Lord Almighty said:

إِنَّا خَلَقْنَا ٱلْإِنسَـٰنَ مِن نُّطْفَةٍ أَمْشَاجٍ نَّبْتَلِيهِ فَجَعَلْنَـٰهُ سَمِيعًا بَصِيرًا

Indeed, We created man from a drop of mixed fluids, in order to test him. So, We gave him hearing and sight.[2]

And He said:

وَجَعَلْنَا بَعْضَكُمْ لِبَعْضٍ فِتْنَةً أَتَصْبِرُونَ وَكَانَ رَبُّكَ بَصِيرًا

We have made some of you as a trial for others. Will you have patience? For your Lord is All-Seeing.[3]

---

[2] Al-Insan: 2
[3] Al-Furqan: 20

And He said:

لِّنَفْتِنَهُمْ فِيهِ وَمَن يُعْرِضْ عَن ذِكْرِ رَبِّهِ يَسْلُكْهُ عَذَابًا صَعَدًا

*As a test for them. But whoever turns away from the re-
membrance of his Lord, He will make him suffer an ardu-
ous punishment.*[4]

Truly, this pandemic is a great trial, as the Almighty
said:

أَوَلَا يَرَوْنَ أَنَّهُمْ يُفْتَنُونَ فِى كُلِّ عَامٍ مَّرَّةً أَوْ مَرَّتَيْنِ ثُمَّ لَا
يَتُوبُونَ وَلَا هُمْ يَذَّكَّرُونَ

*Do they not see that they are put to trial once or twice
every year? Yet they neither repent, nor do they take
heed.*[5]

Therefore, we must, as in every trial, hold ourselves
accountable, appraise our behavior and way of life, and re-
form whatever was corrupted of us.

2. Is it a punishment?

Everything that occurs in this world is by the command and permission of Allah Almighty. He is the Prudent
Creator. He said:

لَهُ مَا فِى ٱلسَّمَـٰوَٰتِ وَمَا فِى ۞ ٱلرَّحْمَـٰنُ عَلَى ٱلْعَرْشِ ٱسْتَوَىٰ
ٱلْأَرْضِ وَمَا بَيْنَهُمَا وَمَا تَحْتَ ٱلثَّرَىٰ

*The Most Compassionate rose over the Throne. To Him
belongs all that is in the heavens and all that is on earth,*

---

[4] Al-Jinn: 17
[5] Al-Tawbah: 126

and all that is between them, and all that is beneath the soil.[6]

Therefore, the main question is: Is our Lord Almighty furious with humanity because they misbehaved in creation and corrupted nature to the extent that corruption has spread on land and sea, as the Almighty said:

ظَهَرَ ٱلْفَسَادُ فِى ٱلْبَرِّ وَٱلْبَحْرِ بِمَا كَسَبَتْ أَيْدِى ٱلنَّاسِ لِيُذِيقَهُم بَعْضَ ٱلَّذِى عَمِلُواْ لَعَلَّهُمْ يَرْجِعُونَ

Corruption has spread on land and sea as a result of what people's hands have done, so that Allah may cause them to taste (the consequences of) some of their deeds and perhaps they might return (to the Right Path).[7]

They have wronged themselves to the furthest degrees. A small insignificant minority have confiscated the rights of most of the world and wasted their resources in developing weapons of mass destruction which threaten to end life on earth. The laws ruling the world today are crueler than the laws of the jungle in conflicts and spreading fear. Our Lord said:

قُلْ هُوَ ٱلْقَادِرُ عَلَىٰٓ أَن يَبْعَثَ عَلَيْكُمْ عَذَابًا مِّن فَوْقِكُمْ أَوْ مِن تَحْتِ أَرْجُلِكُمْ أَوْ يَلْبِسَكُمْ شِيَعًا وَيُذِيقَ بَعْضَكُم بَأْسَ بَعْضٍ ٱنظُرْ كَيْفَ نُصَرِّفُ ٱلْآيَٰتِ لَعَلَّهُمْ يَفْقَهُونَ

Say, "He is Capable to send a punishment from above you or from beneath your feet, or split you into factions, and make you suffer at the hands of one another." See how We diversify the signs, so that they may understand.[8]

---

[6] Taha: 5-6
[7] Al-Rum: 41
[8] Al-Anam: 65

We ask once again: Is this pandemic a dire punishment due to our Lord's wrath on us? Or is it a mere reminder of what is worst? Surely, our Lord has tested us with this pandemic to remind us in hope that we return to the right path and fix our problems. In which case, our responsibilities have greatly increased to face our points of weakness. The Almighty said:

وَلَنُذِيقَنَّهُم مِّنَ ٱلْعَذَابِ ٱلْأَدْنَىٰ دُونَ ٱلْعَذَابِ ٱلْأَكْبَرِ لَعَلَّهُمْ يَرْجِعُونَ

We will certainly make them taste some minor punishment prior to the greater punishment, so that they may return.[9]

Therefore, the purpose is to alert us to that which threatens to destroy civilization if not fixed seriously and urgently.

3. Isolation and Distancing

When the doctors recommended people to self-isolate and practice social distancing, the community split into those who complied with it, willingly and unwillingly, and those who disregarded it. Truly, it was a pioneering experiment in the depth of human culture and their awareness. We discovered [through it], the need for more knowledge, and that media (despite its plenitude) was incapable of delivering facts to the people.

On the other hand, we see that a group of believers willingly followed the orders of the religious leadership, and complied with what the specialists advised, seeking nearness to Allah Almighty and in fear of His punishment. Thus, we were able to see the extent of people's need for religion.

---

[9] Al-Sajdah: 21

4. Home Isolation

Many isolated themselves at home and benefitted by this isolation in several ways:

a. Some people took the opportunity for solitude to become closer to their Merciful, Beneficent Lord, by reciting His Noble Book, reading the narrated supplications, and completing their missed prayers or fasting days.

b. Some discovered that they have a kind family, as they had an opportunity to get to know them better and realized how much they had lost when they only used their family to fulfill their urgent materialistic needs.

c. Others contemplated about themselves and discovered their points of weakness and shallowness of their knowledge. So, they began reading books and participating in cultural seminars and courses, especially those regarding religious awareness and Islamic culture.

d. Other people's contemplation of life led them to fix their way of life, protecting them [from such trials] in the future God-willing.

Mohammed Taqi al-Modarresi
The Holy City of Karbala
11 of the Blessed month of Ramadan 1441 AH

Part 1

The Rulings of Health and Safety

Preface

Good life is a value of faith, and one of its foundations is wellness. Achieving it would be through protection, treatment, and peace of mind. Examples of protection are refraining from evil, purification, and avoiding extravagance in food and drink, rejecting wrong, and choosing good. Examples of treatment are fasting, prayer, pilgrimage, and seeking cure with honey. Peace of mind, as well, protects the human being from many illnesses and helps cure others.

The Rulings of Health

It seems from the [religious] texts that faith promotes good life, and one of its implementations is wellness. There are many degrees of wellness, some of which are obligatory to be met and kept, while others are recommended. They are as follows:

a. The lowest degree of wellness is that which protects one's life and organs, and it is obligatory.

b. The degree which protects the person from the risk of harm which results in public weakness, for example, or a great harm in one's capabilities, such as vision, hearing, speech, or sexual abilities. It may also be obligatory.

c. The degree which protects public wellness, and abandoning it causes great corruption, such as the spread of deadly diseases, and it is obligatory.

d. The degree which protects the community from viruses that may result in the death of only some people due to health complications, such as protecting the environment from influenza. This may be obligatory in some cases as well.

e. The highest degree of health protection is that which guarantees safety from all kinds of illnesses. It is recommended unless it is made obligatory by the religious authority.

Below are the details of all five degrees:

Protecting One's Life and Organs

The Holy Quran

1.

يَـٰٓأَيُّهَا ٱلَّذِينَ ءَامَنُواْ ٱسْتَجِيبُواْ لِلَّهِ وَلِلرَّسُولِ إِذَا دَعَاكُمْ لِمَا يُحْيِيكُمْ وَٱعْلَمُوٓاْ أَنَّ ٱللَّهَ يَحُولُ بَيْنَ ٱلْمَرْءِ وَقَلْبِهِ وَأَنَّهُ إِلَيْهِ تُحْشَرُونَ

O' you who have believed, respond to Allah and to the Messenger when he calls you to that which gives you life. And know that Allah intervenes between a man and his heart and that to Him you will be gathered.[10]

2.

وَمِنْهُم مَّن يَقُولُ رَبَّنَآ ءَاتِنَا فِى ٱلدُّنْيَا حَسَنَةً وَفِى ٱلْـَٔاخِرَةِ حَسَنَةً وَقِنَا عَذَابَ ٱلنَّارِ

Yet there are others who say, "Our Lord! Grant us the good of this world and the Hereafter and protect us from the torment of the Fire."[11]

3.

---

[10] Al-Anfal: 24
[11] Al-Baqarah: 201

يَـٰٓأَيُّهَا ٱلَّذِينَ ءَامَنُواْ لَا تَأْكُلُوٓاْ أَمْوَٰلَكُم بَيْنَكُم بِٱلْبَـٰطِلِ إِلَّآ أَن تَكُونَ تِجَـٰرَةً عَن تَرَاضٍ مِّنكُمْ وَلَا تَقْتُلُوٓاْ أَنفُسَكُمْ إِنَّ ٱللَّهَ كَانَ بِكُمْ رَحِيمًا

O' you who have believed, do not consume one another's wealth unjustly but only trade by mutual consent. And do not kill yourselves [or one another]. Indeed, Allah is to you ever Merciful.[12]

4.

وَأَنفِقُواْ فِى سَبِيلِ ٱللَّهِ وَلَا تُلْقُواْ بِأَيْدِيكُمْ إِلَى ٱلتَّهْلُكَةِ وَأَحْسِنُوٓاْ إِنَّ ٱللَّهَ يُحِبُّ ٱلْمُحْسِنِينَ

Spend in the cause of Allah and do not let your own hands throw you into destruction. And do good, for Allah certainly loves the good-doers.[13]

5.

مَنْ عَمِلَ صَـٰلِحًا مِّن ذَكَرٍ أَوْ أُنثَىٰ وَهُوَ مُؤْمِنٌ فَلَنُحْيِيَنَّهُۥ حَيَوٰةً طَيِّبَةً وَلَنَجْزِيَنَّهُمْ أَجْرَهُم بِأَحْسَنِ مَا كَانُواْ يَعْمَلُونَ

Whoever does good, whether male or female, and is a believer, We will surely bless them with a good life, and We will certainly reward them according to the best of their deeds.[14]

Insight into the Revelation

1. The true religion has called to a good life, and our Lord has ordered us to answer His Messenger when he calls us to what gives us life, the call of the righteous, as well, was to a good life in the world and the hereafter. The means for

---

[12] Al-Nisa: 29
[13] Al-Baqarah: 195
[14] Al-Nahl: 97

it are righteous deeds, and health is a condition for that good life.

2. On the other hand, protecting oneself and preserving life is a natural obligation which the religion has placed multitudes of rulings and manners to achieve. We are not here to list these rulings, but we will refer to the most important ones below.

The Rulings

1. There is no doubt that destroying life, killing a soul, and damaging organs or physical capabilities is a forbidden act religiously.

2. This inviolability encompasses the causes which result in it, such as intentional negligence which results in death, or damages an organ or ability, or committing suicide.

3. The impermissibility of throwing oneself into destruction may mean protecting it to the extent necessary. So, whoever fails to protect himself despite while being capable and knowledgeable of doing so, to the extent that people consider him "destroying himself" has committed a sin.

4. Based on the obligation of protecting oneself, it is obligatory to follow the health regulations to the extent which protects life from destruction and protects parts, organs, and abilities from damage.

5. There are several impermissible acts which the religion has explained to be impermissible due to their harm on human life or health. Therefore, it is obligatory to avoid such acts.

6. A person must manage his personal life in detail and with wisdom. He should pay attention to his food and drink, sleep schedule, and activities. He should pay attention to his strength, fitness, and health. He should also maintain the soundness of his mind and nerves. He must give his body its share of pleasure and comfort. To achieve all of this, every human must have comprehensive knowledge of life; what is good, what benefits him, and what harms him.

7. Everyone should impose on themselves strict health regulations, including: Caring about cleanliness, avoiding germs and viruses, visiting doctors when necessary, and precision when following their orders.

8. Society should care about its members, especially the upcoming generation. It should provide all the necessary means for the safety of their bodies and nerves.

9. Jurisprudents determine rulings based on the general concepts of the religion.

10. Countries should strengthen surveillance in matters regarding causes of destruction, such as car accidents, labor risks, sport risks, and their likes.

Health and Severe Harm

The Noble Tradition

1. It has been narrated from Imam al-Sadiq ('a): *"Any type of seed which is nutritional to the human body and strength is permissible to eat, and anything which is harmful for the human body is impermissible to eat, except in necessities."*[15]

---

[15] Al-Anfal: 24

2. In the infamous narration from the Prophet: *"Harm may neither be inflicted nor reciprocated in Islam."*[16]

3. Ibn Idrees said in his book *al-Sara'ir*: It has been narrated from the Messenger of Allah (s) and the Imams from his progeny to seek treatment, they said: *"Seek treatment, as Allah has not placed a disease without providing its cure."*[17]

The Rulings

1. There are some types of illnesses that may not result in death or immediate harm to an organ or ability, but may result in great damage, such as diabetes, or any long-term illness. It may not result in death, but it is known to cause great harm to the individual. It seems that protecting oneself from such diseases is obligatory.

2. It is more obligatory to seek treatment from such diseases, if neglecting it is considered destruction of oneself.

Public Health and Corruption

The Holy Quran

وَأَنفِقُواْ فِى سَبِيلِ ٱللَّهِ وَلَا تُلْقُواْ بِأَيْدِيكُمْ إِلَى ٱلتَّهْلُكَةِ وَأَحْسِنُوٓاْ إِنَّ ٱللَّهَ يُحِبُّ ٱلْمُحْسِنِينَ

Spend in the cause of Allah and do not let your own hands throw you into destruction. And do good, for Allah certainly loves the good-doers.[18]

---

[16] Man La Yahdhuruhu al-Faqih, vol. 4, p. 334, n. 5818.
[17] Bihar al-Anwar, v. 59, p. 65, following narration 9.
[18] Al-Baqarah: 195

مَنْ عَمِلَ صَلِحًا مِّن ذَكَرٍ أَوْ أُنثَىٰ وَهُوَ مُؤْمِنٌ فَلَنُحْيِيَنَّهُۥ حَيَوٰةً طَيِّبَةً
وَلَنَجْزِيَنَّهُمْ أَجْرَهُم بِأَحْسَنِ مَا كَانُوا يَعْمَلُونَ

Whoever does good, whether male or female, and is a believer, We will surely bless them with a good life, and We will certainly reward them according to the best of their deeds.[19]

Insight into the Revelation

Allah Almighty very strictly forbids spreading corruption on Earth. Avoiding greater corruption is considered a way to limit the guardianship of the unbelievers. Therefore, it is obligatory to prevent the spread of corruption in all its forms. One of these forms, is giving importance to public health to protect the people from harm and corruption.

The Rulings

1. It is important to prevent the circulation of spoiled foods, and to supervise the producers and sellers on all levels, from farmers to factories to restaurants and bakeries, as well as grinders, butchers, and their likes.

2. It is also very important to monitor the water sources, rivers, reservoirs, pumps, and pipes, to preserve them from contamination of microbes, radioactive materials, or other harmful materials.

3. It is obligatory to protect against deadly viruses with vaccinations and to prevent their spread from infected areas to safe areas.

---

[19] Al-Nahl: 97

4. It is necessary to impose health regulations in schools, workplaces, factories, and other places of gathering to prevent the spread of viruses.

5. It is also necessary to provide shelters to quarantine those who are infected with infectious diseases, such as smallpox, leprosy, TB, AIDS, COVID-19, and their likes, to protect others from becoming infected.

6. It is important to regulate marriages to prevent the spread of dangerous STDs, and to protect the offspring from genetic diseases.

Public Health and Good Life

The Holy Quran

ٱلَّذِينَ يَتَّبِعُونَ ٱلرَّسُولَ ٱلنَّبِيَّ ٱلْأُمِّيَّ ٱلَّذِى يَجِدُونَهُ مَكْتُوبًا عِندَهُمْ فِى ٱلتَّوْرَىٰةِ وَٱلْإِنجِيلِ يَأْمُرُهُم بِٱلْمَعْرُوفِ وَيَنْهَىٰهُمْ عَنِ ٱلْمُنكَرِ وَيُحِلُّ لَهُمُ ٱلطَّيِّبَٰتِ وَيُحَرِّمُ عَلَيْهِمُ ٱلْخَبَٰئِثَ وَيَضَعُ عَنْهُمْ إِصْرَهُمْ وَٱلْأَغْلَٰلَ ٱلَّتِى كَانَتْ عَلَيْهِمْ فَٱلَّذِينَ ءَامَنُوا۟ بِهِ وَعَزَّرُوهُ وَنَصَرُوهُ وَٱتَّبَعُوا۟ ٱلنُّورَ ٱلَّذِى أُنزِلَ مَعَهُ أُو۟لَٰئِكَ هُمُ ٱلْمُفْلِحُونَ

Those who follow the Messenger – the unlettered Prophet – whose description they find in their Torah and the Gospel. He enjoins them to do what is good and forbids them from what is evil; he makes lawful for them what is pure and makes unlawful for them from what is impure; he relieves them of their burden and the shackles that were on them. So those who believe in him, they honor and support him, and follow the light which is sent down with him – it is they who will be successful. "[20]

---

[20] Al-Araf: 157

وَٱلرُّجْزَ فَٱهْجُرْ ● وَثِيَابَكَ فَطَهِّرْ

And your clothing purify. And uncleanliness avoid.[21]

إِنَّ ٱللَّهَ يُحِبُّ ٱلتَّوَّبِينَ وَيُحِبُّ ٱلْمُتَطَهِّرِينَ

Allah loves those who frequently repent and He loves those who purify themselves.[22]

Insight into the Revelation

1. Our Lord has forbidden what is impure because it causes diseases. Carrion, swine, alcohol, and all that which harms you of food and drink are enemies of your health.

2. He has forbidden shameful acts, both openly and in secret, because they harm our health. He has also commanded us to avoid impurity, to seek purity, and to purify ourselves in specific times, to maintain our health.

The Rulings

1. Religious teaching forbid impurities, recommend purity in all its levels, and consider cleanliness a value of faith which every human should observe based on his ability.

2. Society should fight contamination in all its forms. That is why there must be strict, comprehensive regulations on all public facilities to maintain cleanliness from all kinds of germs.

3. Governments must prevent infectious diseases from entering their country, as well as unhealthy foods.

---

[21] Al-Muddathir: 4-5
[22] Al-Baqarah: 222

The Highest degree of Individual health

The Noble Tradition

1. The Commander of Faithful ('a) said: *"Well-being is the most pleasant of blessings,"*[23] and he said: *"Well-being is the most noble of garments."*[24] He also said: *"The pleasure of life is in well-being."*[25]

2. He ('a) said: *"Health is the best of blessings,"*[26] and: *"Health completes pleasure,"*[27] and: *"Bliss in this life is safety and physical health, and the complete bliss in the afterlife is entering heaven."*[28]

The Rulings

1. It is recommended for a person to maintain the highest standards of well-being. He should seek to have his blood pressure, diet, abilities, heart rate, etc. in the best medical standards.

2. It is recommended for a person to protect himself from all impurities, maintain a good diet, and to observe a fitness routine.

3. Generally, Islam has encouraged health as an essential value. There are narrated religious texts which give many teachings that benefit health. It ranges from choosing the partner in marital life, the manners of sex, pregnancy, nutritious diets during pregnancy, and breastfeeding, to the

---

[23] Oyoun al-Hikam w al-Mawa'idh, p. 31, n. 504.
[24] Ghurar al-Hikam w Durar al-Kalim, p. 88, n. 1693.
[25] Oyoun al-Hikam w al-Mawa'idh, p. 188, n. 3854.
[26] Ibid, p. 23, n. 177.
[27] Ibid, p. 186, n. 3771.
[28] Ma'ani al-Akhbar, p. 408.

manners of food, drink, sleep, bath, etc. Together, with the will of Allah, these manners extend the human's life and protect his body and abilities.

4. It is recommended to pray to Allah asking for good health, as all things are under the command of Allah Almighty. The prayer of Ali Ibn al-Hussain ('a) for well-being was: *"O' Allah, send Your blessings upon Mohammed and his progeny, and make me well with a sufficient healing, exalted growing well-being. A well-being that will cause further well-being in my body. A well-being in this life and the afterlife. And bless me with health, security, and safety in my religion and body."[29]*

5. Because health is such an important value, we must give serious importance to it by implementing the following teachings:

a. To regulate prevention systems in the country to the best of our ability, especially systems regulating food, drink, and materials used in them. As well as regulation and safety regarding products.

b. Social health awareness which seeks to teach the individual at least the basic standards of well-being, understanding his abilities, how to protect himself from diseases, how to increase his immunity with food, drink, and fitness. As well as knowing the different diseases, their causes, and how to prevent and cure them. This awareness should be raised in schools, from elementary classes to higher degrees, as well as in visual and audible media.

---

[29] Imam al-Sajjad ('a) prayer when he asked Allah for well-being, al-Sahifa al-Sajjadiyah, s. 23.

c. Providing doctors, nurses, medications, hospitals, clinics, and all forms of healthcare for every human is a natural right.

d. Jurisprudents should issue religious rulings regarding specific important health issues, such as obliging vaccinations during a deadly pandemic after consulting experts and specialists.

e. Good doers should provide healthcare services [to those who are unable to afford it] for the sake of Allah Almighty.

f. All members of society should contribute to the fight against health corruption when the nation is challenged with a dangerous health calamity, such as deadly viruses.

Health is a Human Right

The Holy Quran

يَـٰٓأَيُّهَا ٱلنَّاسُ إِنَّا خَلَقْنَـٰكُم مِّن ذَكَرٍ وَأُنثَىٰ وَجَعَلْنَـٰكُمْ شُعُوبًا وَقَبَآئِلَ لِتَعَارَفُوٓاْ إِنَّ أَكْرَمَكُمْ عِندَ ٱللَّهِ أَتْقَىٰكُمْ إِنَّ ٱللَّهَ عَلِيمٌ خَبِيرٌ

O' mankind, We have created you from a male and a female, and made you into nations and tribes so that you may recognize one another. Indeed, the most noble of you before Allah is the most righteous among you. Indeed, Allah is All-Knowing, All-Aware.[30]

It appears that the 'recognition' mentioned in the verse means to accept each other's rights, and of course the most important of rights is the right of life. From it, other

---

[30] Al-Muddathir: 4-5

rights branch out, such as the right of security, safety, comfort (in food, drink, shelter, etc.), and the right of health.

The Noble Tradition

The Messenger of Allah (s) said: *"The one who does not care about Muslims is not one of them, and he who hears a man calling: O' Muslims and does not answer him is not a Muslim."*[31]

Insight into the Revelation

1. The right of life is the root of all other rights. Health and physical safety are essentials of life.

2. The texts which encouraged charity, included charity to those who are physically incapable.

3. The texts that stressed the importance of Muslims caring about one another include caring about providing them with the necessary healthcare.

4. We can interpret from the different texts that supporting each other in the matter of health is very important to the best of our ability and depending on the necessity.

5. Therefore, healthcare is a goal which both people and governments should seek to provide for everyone along with the available means.

6. Legislators should also seek to place laws which provide everyone with this right, God-willing.

---

[31] Al-Kafi, v. 2, p. 164.

Part 2
Rulings Regarding How to Deal the Coronavirus

1. Following the health guidance

Question: The Ministry of Health, in accordance with the WHO, released detailed and varied guidance regarding COVID-19 precaution and prevention. This guidance includes individual behavior, social relations, and how to act in markets, public transit, travel, and so on. So, what is our religious duty regarding such matters?

Answer: If the spread of the disease is quick and serious to the extent that it threatens public health and community safety, and results in great numbers of cases and deaths, following such instructions is a religious obligation to protect oneself from disease and not cause harm to others. Our Lord, the Almighty, said:

وَلَا تُلْقُواْ بِأَيْدِيكُمْ إِلَى ٱلتَّهْلُكَةِ

And do not let your own hands throw you into destruction.[32]

And in a noble narration, which is considered a jurisprudential principle, the Messenger (s) says: *"Harm may neither be inflicted nor reciprocated in Islam."*[33]

2. Mandatory and voluntary quarantine

Question: In our area, the government enforced on travelers from the EU and USA which have been plagued by the virus mandatory health quarantine in special facilities and hospitals until they are proven to be safe from the virus.

---

[32] Al-Baqarah: 195
[33] Man La Yahdhuruhu al-Faqih, vol. 4, p. 334, n. 5818.

Is it obligatory for the traveler to follow this requirement? If he can avoid it in any way, would it be permissible?

Answer: If the likelihood of catching or carrying this virus is rational, it is obligatory to comply with the quarantine to protect oneself and the community.

Question: What does rational likelihood mean? Who is considered rational in such matters?

Answer: What is meant by rational is the specialists in every field. So, regarding the disease, the opinion of doctors and health centers is what should be followed. Therefore, the 'likelihood' determined by them is what should be met and taken seriously.

3. The debtor who is unable to pay

Question: Due to quarantine and health lockdowns, many markets have closed, buying, and selling goods has become obstructed, and therefore many people have become unemployed and face financial issues. Most importantly, they have become unable to pay their debts in the required times. So, what is the ruling regarding a debtor who is unable to pay? What should the creditor do?

Answer:
a. It is obligatory for the financially capable debtor to pay his debt on time, whether it is an immediate or deferred debt.

b. If the debtor can pay, and the time of the debt has come, it is impermissible for him to procrastinate in payment. In fact, it is considered a great sin.

c. If the debtor is insolvent or unable to pay (like in the case of many debtors currently), it is impermissible for the creditor to pressure him into paying and to coerce him by constantly asking. It is obligatory for him to give him enough time until he can pay. The Almighty says:

وَإِن كَانَ ذُو عُسْرَةٍ فَنَظِرَةٌ إِلَىٰ مَيْسَرَةٍ وَأَن تَصَدَّقُواْ خَيْرٌ لَّكُمْ إِن كُنتُمْ تَعْلَمُونَ

If it is difficult for someone to repay a debt, postpone it until a time of ease. And if you waive it as an act of charity, it will be better for you, if only you knew.[34]

And in the noble narration from Imam al-Sadiq ('a), he says: *"Our father, the Messenger of Allah (s) used to say: It is not [permissible] for a Muslim to force another insolvent Muslim [into paying]. Whoever gives time to an insolvent, Allah shades him with His shadow in the Day in which there is no shade but His."*[35]

4. The Fasting of those infected with COVID-19 or those who fear infection

Question: We are entering the blessed month of Ramadan, and the COVID-19 virus continues to spread in different areas. Some recommend to constantly drink water in order to reduce the risk of catching this dangerous virus, because not drinking much water, according to this claim, decreases immunity, and mouth dryness allows the virus to enter into the respiratory system if it enters the mouth. While drinking water helps bring it down to the stomach which destroys it. So, is permissible for Muslims not to fast in the month of Ramadan this year for this reason?

---

[34] Al-Baqarah: 280
[35] al-Kafi, vol. 8, p. 9.

Answer: The infected person who breaks his fast should fast some other days, and his ruling is that of an ill person.

As for the healthy person who fears infection from fasting or finds it very difficult with the current circumstances, he should avoid places of infection and meet all the precautionary conditions even home quarantine to be able to complete his obligation of fasting. The mentioned recommendations, if they are true, are for those in places of high risk of infection.

Therefore, it is obligatory for the Muslims to observe fasting. However, there is a ruling for every Muslim depending on the rational degree of fear from infection while observing all the preventive and precautionary measures [which he decides].

5. The Pilgrimage of the infected and those who fear infection

Question: Someone is capable of pilgrimage and had planned to perform it this year, but the spread of the virus made him hesitant out of fear of infection, especially because he has diabetes and High Blood Pressure which increases the risk of infection. Is it obligatory for him to perform the pilgrimage despite all of this?

Answer: One of the conditions of capability is physical capability which is required for the pilgrimage. This means not being ill with an illness which prevents the pilgrim from performing his travel for pilgrimage or makes it difficult on him to an extent which he cannot stand, or fear of infection from a deadly virus due to gathering. Therefore, the ill who is unable to go to the Sacred House of Allah or finds it extremely difficult, is not required to perform the pilgrimage even if he has all the other conditions which make it obligatory. He should wait till he becomes better or till life returns to normal, to perform his pilgrimage safely God-willing.

It has been narrated from Abdullah Ibn al-Hajjaj that he said: *I asked Abu Abdullah ('a) about the Almighty's saying [Pilgrimage to this House is an obligation by Allah upon whoever is able among the people], he said (regarding the meaning of ability): "Health in his body, and ability in his money."*[36]

6. If governments prevent traveling to the Holy Lands

Question: If the virus continues to spread and is unable to be contained around the world, especially in the Arabian Peninsula, in which the government suffers to manage the health of two million pilgrims, is it permissible for Islamic governments to prevent its citizens from traveling for the pilgrimages of Hajj and Umrah?

Answer: If public interest requires this, with the recommendations of trusted experts and specialists, it is permissible. In fact, it may be obligatory in cases of extreme danger to the community.

7. Not shaking hands due to fear of infection

Question: If someone shakes my hand or extends his hand for a handshake, and I do not shake his hand because it is a primary way of infection, is this considered disrespectful?

Answer: With fear of harm from the handshake, it should be avoided. Not engaging in a handshake with one

---

[36] Tafsir al-Ayyashi, vol. 1, p. 193, n.117.

who extends their hand would not be considered disrespectful.

8. Evading Quarantine

Question: Some countries require travelers coming
from countries with high cases to quarantine. I am a busi-
nessman, and my business will be affected if I am quaran-
tined. So, can I travel to another country, as a transit, to by-
pass the quarantine?

Answer: Evading quarantine with fear of transmit-
ting the virus to others is impermissible.

9. Covering up the infection

Question: Some countries prevent their citizens from
going to the holy shrines, and whoever does, is prevented
from travel for a whole year. If the visitor is infected with
COVID-19, is it permissible to hide his infection?

Answer: With the risk of harming others by transmit-
ting the virus, it is precautionary to not cover it up.

10. Using alcoholic disinfectants and antiseptics

Question: Some disinfectants have 70% alcohol, are
they permissible to use?

Answer: There is no issue with using these alcoholic
disinfectants given that the alcohol is of a synthetic, non-or-
ganic, source. Not knowing their source is sufficient (for per-
missibility).

11. Reporting an infection

Question: If a family member is infected or suspected of infection, is it obligatory to inform the health facilities?

Answer: It is recommended, rather precautionary (obligatory) to inform the competent authorities to avoid the harm caused by ignoring the virus.

12. Preparing the dead during the virus

Question: The World Health Organization protocols state to not wash the corpse of a person who passed away with the virus, and to bury him in a graveyard designated for covid victims to prevent the spread of the virus. Is it obligatory to follow these protocols, such as not washing the body and burying in designated areas?

Answer: If possible, it obligatory to perform all burial ceremonies which do not cause the spread of the virus. As for burial, there is no problem in burying them in designated areas.

13. Violating the will of burying in a specific place

Question: If a person infected with the COVID-19 virus requests to be buried in a specific place in his will, is it obligatory to follow his will?

Answer: It is not obligatory to follow the will of burying in a specific place when fearing the spread of the virus.

14. Monopoly of medical supplies

Question: I am a pharmacist. Some people come to me asking for large numbers of (virus) prevention supplies. This will harm others as there will not be many supplies and they would be very high-priced. Therefore, is it permissible for me to sell him more than his need?

Answer: If you know that the person is buying the virus prevention supplies for monopoly, it is impermissible to sell him it.

15. Not working due to the virus

Question: I am a healthcare employee. I agreed with my co-workers, and with the permission of my employer, to not go to work because I have a chronic disease which makes me more likely to catch the coronavirus, what is the ruling of the salary I am paid?

Answer: If this does not violate the government and company guidelines, there is no problem.

16. Religious dues for virus treatment

Question: Is it permissible for us to spend some of our religious dues through specialized institutes to cure coronavirus patients?

Answer: It is permissible to spend some of the religious dues to fight the coronavirus or to help the sick.

17. Prayers to defend against the virus

Question: Some prayers are circulated throughout social media to defend against the virus, is it permissible to share these prayers?

Answer: Any prayer which does not contradict the foundations of faith is permissible to recite and share, not with the intention of being narrated from the Infallibles ('a), but rather with the intention to come closer [to Allah].

18. Visiting the shrines with masks and gloves

Question: Is it right to require visitors of the holy shrines to wear masks and gloves to prevent the spread of the virus and infections.

Answer: If public benefit requires that, there is no problem with it.

19. Disinfecting the shrines, mosques, and centers

Question: Is it permissible to disinfect the mosques, shrines, and centers with disinfectants? Does that not contradict the holiness of these places?

Answer: It is permissible and there is no contradiction, especially when it is to prevent the causes of the virus to maintain their sanctity. In fact, it may be considered a kind of purification which Allah ordered when He (swt) said:

أَن طَهِّرَا بَيْتِيَ لِلطَّآئِفِينَ وَٱلْعَٰكِفِينَ وَٱلرُّكَّعِ ٱلسُّجُودِ

"Purify My House for those who perform circulation and those who are staying [there] for worship and those who bow and prostrate [in prayer]."[37]

20. Closing shrines, mosques, and centers

Question: What do you think of the decision made by some Islamic governments to close mosques, shrines, and centers, or to place restrictions on visitors or worshippers?

---

[37] Al-Baqarah: 280

Answer: If it is to protect the safety of the people and to prevent the spread of the virus caused by gatherings and neglecting social distancing, there is no problem in it. But we advise these governments to provide the viral precaution supplies, then to re-open these places of worship.

21. Gathering for events

Question: Experts and specialists say that one can get infected with the virus through other infected people, and that the virus may move from one person to another through small particles dispersed when sneezing or coughing. These particles then settle on surfaces surrounding other people. Then, others may become infected with the virus by touching these items and then touching their eyes, nose, or mouth. A person may also become infected if they breathe in these infected particles. Therefore, it is very important to be at least one meter (3 feet) away from an infected person.

For this reason, governments have prohibited all kinds of gatherings (for happy and sad occasions, mosques, universities, as well as markets, halls, and all other places of gathering). Therefore:

a. Is it permissible for us not to follow these regulations?

Answer: If neglecting these regulations causes the spread of the virus, it is not permissible.

b. Is it permissible for someone infected with the virus, who may infect others, to refuse quarantine and attend these gatherings?

Answer: It is impermissible to cause oneself to be infected with a deadly virus. It is also impermissible to cause others to become infected.

c. If an infected person neglected the precautionary guidelines which prevent the spread of the coronavirus, and caused the infection of others, or even their death, what is his ruling?

Answer: His ruling is that of a trustee [meaning if he had neglected it intentionally, he must pay the diyya] if he is proven to be the cause.

22. Unemployment

Question: As you know, there were many workers and small business owners who were affected by the nation-wide lockdown, some who even became unemployed due to the closing of markets, factories, and trade. Are such people considered needy?

Answer: Anyone who is unable to ensure his or his family's needs for one year (physically or realistically) is considered needy. Therefore, believers who can help him meet his needs, will be rewarded greatly for doing so.

23. Credit from usurious banks

Question: In the current circumstances (the spread of the virus and imminence of financial issues), is it permissible to borrow money from usurious (interest-taking) banks to maintain life necessities, especially when there aren't Islamic banks to loan from?

Answer: Usurious loans (whether from banks or individuals) are impermissible expect in necessities (as necessities permit forbidden acts), yet one must limit himself to necessities.

24. Congregational prayers during the pandemic

Question: One of the primary causes of the spread of the coronavirus is gathering. Specialized institutes have recommended to observe social distancing. Therefore, is it permissible to perform congregational prayers with a distance of one meter and half or two meters between one person and another?

Answer: It is impermissible due to the difficulty of meeting the conditions of connection.

25. Kin relations during the pandemic

Question: What is the opinion of your eminence regarding to decrease in kin relations and even marital relations during the pandemic? Isn't cutting ties with kin impermissible?

Answer: In the current exceptional and urgent circumstances, one must observe both matters. That is by following the safety precautions on one hand, while limiting kin relations on the other to the least degree of obligation using modern social media tools and delaying direct unnecessary visits till after the pandemic God-willing.

26. Refuge to the lands of non-believers in fear of the virus

Question: Is it permissible to immigrate from our Islamic land to the land of non-believers in fear of infection from the coronavirus?

Answer: In theory, it is permissible if you preserve your faith and meet your religious rituals. Although, in these current exceptional circumstances (the COVID-19 pandemic), the land of non-believers has become more dangerous and less safe health-wise than Islamic lands.

27. Contracts and financial obligations

Question: The spread of the coronavirus caused the closing of most trade activities, as well as import and export. This delayed many financial obligations and contracts, so what is the religious ruling regarding this?

Answer: Everyone must cooperate and harmonize in these matters in which contractors are unable to fulfill their contracts due to the current exceptional circumstances.

28. Obeying tyrants regarding the pandemic

Question: If a ruler is unjust and rules against what Allah has commanded, is it obligatory to obey him in the orders given regarding precaution from the spread of the coronavirus?

Answer: The guidelines for the prevention of the spread of the virus are guidelines which religious teachings endorse before any local government or global organization. Therefore, obeying these guidelines is obeying Allah, not the tyrant.